Nutritious
APPETITE

Your Complete Manual
To Lose Excessive Fat
The Healthy Way

Michelle R. Paschke

Table of Content

Nutritious APPETITE

Introduction

A sound eating routine is an eating regimen that keeps up with or works on generally wellbeing. A solid eating routine gives the body fundamental sustenance: liquid, macronutrients, for example, protein, micronutrients like nutrients, and sufficient fiber and food energy.

A sound eating routine might contain natural products, vegetables, and entire grains, and may incorporate next to zero handled food or improved refreshments. The prerequisites for a sound eating routine can be met from an assortment of plant-based and creature based food sources, albeit extra wellsprings of vitamin B12 are required for those following a veggie lover diet. Different nourishment guides are distributed by clinical and legislative organizations to teach people on the thing they ought to eat to be solid. Nourishment realities names are additionally required in certain nations to permit purchasers to pick between food sources in light of the parts pertinent to wellbeing.

CHAPTER ONE

You Are What You Eat

You don't need to be a nutritionist to realize that an eating regimen too high in quick food sources, overabundance sugar and red meat conveys with it a gamble of corpulence and illness like type 2 diabetes and coronary illness.

Garbage like handled or broiled food, candy, pop or business heated products has been deprived of any dietary benefit. So despite the fact that they could assuage your cravings for food they don't give the fundamental nourishment your body needs. They most likely don't leave you feeling extremely incredible by the same token! Recall the last time you reveled in a major feast or additional pastries. As you pushed your seat back from the table to unfasten your jeans you might have encountered heartburn, a swelled stomach and felt drained or drowsy.

Then again, quality food varieties, for example, new vegetables, natural products, nuts and entire grains contain a large group of nutritious goodness: nutrients, minerals, fiber, protein and fundamental omega fats, just to give some examples. Your body needs these supplements to work. Food furnishes us with energy and the unrefined substances to do significant physical processes like getting out squander, fighting off ailment and keeping your heart thumping.

The food that you eat ought to continuously cause you to feel your best so you can maintain your own business, raise a family or care for wiped out or old friends and family - or perhaps you're doing every one of the three! While sickness counteraction is unquestionably a significant motivation to eat well, we frequently neglect the more prompt advantages of a sound eating regimen. Here are only a couple of the advantages you could appreciate:

Expanded Energy

Handled garbage and weighty, rich food varieties can dial back your processing, leaving you drained and drowsy. And keeping in mind that caffeine and refined sugar could provide you with a fast impact of energy now, it will leave you with even less energy some other time when you crash - and you will crash.

Counting protein and complex carbs at every feast

or bite - think heated yams with broiled chicken and a plate of mixed greens - will provide you with a supported wellspring of energy that will endure significantly longer, without the high points and low points.

Better Assimilation

Indigestion, blockage, gas and swelling are undesirable side effects connected with eating a lot of some unacceptable kinds of food. Dinners and bites ought to leave you feeling fulfilled, not overstuffed or wiped out to your stomach.

As well as picking entire food varieties, dialing back to eat at a table from a genuine plate and biting each chomp can likewise assist with lightening stomach related upset. It could likewise assist you with eating less as well!

Further developed Rest and State of mind

That sugar or caffeine high I referenced before isn't about

to screw with your energy, it can likewise interfere with your rest and leave you feeling grouchy - that is putting it pleasantly.

You won't get a decent night's rest in the event that your body is attempting to process a day of unhealthy food or you're actually riding a sugar rush. Then in the event that you haven't had sufficient rest you're surely not going to be a beam of daylight. It's an endless loop -

while you're feeling drowsy you might be more disposed to go after sugar or void carbs.

Attempt to drink your most memorable mug of espresso solely after you've had a sound breakfast and unquestionably don't drink energized refreshments after 2:00 pm. In the event that you will have pastry it's smarter to have it at lunch as opposed to supper so you're not making a beeline for bed with raised glucose.

Life is occupied and you can't stand to be overloaded by unfortunate food decisions. Eating a sound, entire food sources diet will assist you with feeling extraordinary today and keeping in mind that forestalling illness tomorrow.

Nutritious APPETITE

CHAPTER TWO

Importance of Nutrition for Dieting

The significance of a fair eating routine can't be underscored enough for a solid way of life. A sound way of life can be accomplished by keeping a reasonable eating regimen and keeping into thought to meet every one of the fundamental supplements expected by the body. A legitimate dinner plan assists with accomplishing ideal body weight and diminishes the gamble of ongoing illnesses like diabetes, cardiovascular and different kinds of malignant growth.

What is a fair eating regimen?

However, what precisely is a fair eating regimen? In basic words, an eating routine offers the supplements to assist your body with working appropriately. The significance of diet lies in the admission of the perfect proportion of calories. Your body gets the right sustenance when you eat a wide assortment of food wealthy in calories like new products of the soil, entire grains, and proteins.

Calories

Calories are a sign of the energy content in the food. When you admission the food, the calories are eaten when you walk, think, or relax. Overall, an individual might expect around 2000 calories every day to keep up with their body weight. By and large, an individual's calories might rely upon their orientation, age, and active work. Additionally, men need a larger number of calories than ladies. Once more, individuals who are more into practicing require more calories in contrast with individuals who don't. It's likewise critical to recall that the wellspring of calories is similarly significant as the sum. Stuffing your food with void calories, for example those that contain no dietary benefit helps in no manner. Void calories can be found in food sources, for example,

- Sugar

- Margarine

- Treats

- Cakes

- Caffeinated drinks

- Frozen yogurt

- Pizza

Significance of a Fair Eating routine

Eating a sound eating routine is tied in with feeling perfect, having more energy, working on your wellbeing, and supporting your state of mind. Great sustenance, actual work, and sound body weight are fundamental pieces of an individual's general wellbeing and prosperity.

There's no scrutinizing the significance of good food in your life. Except if you keep a legitimate eating regimen for a sound body, you might be inclined to illnesses, disease, or even weariness. The significance of nutritious nourishment for kids particularly should be featured since any other way they might turn out to be inclined to a few development and formative issues. Probably the most widely recognized medical issues that emerge from absence of a fair eating regimen are coronary illness, malignant growth, stroke, and diabetes.

Being genuinely dynamic oversees numerous medical conditions and works on emotional wellness by decreasing pressure, discouragement, and torment.

Normal activity assists with forestalling metabolic condition, stroke, hypertension, joint inflammation, and uneasiness.

What falls under a fair eating routine?

A reasonable eating routine incorporates some particular quality nutritional categories under it:

- Vegetables, for example, mixed greens, boring

vegetables, vegetables like beans and peas, red and orange vegetables, and others like eggplant

• Natural products that incorporate entire organic products, new or frozen organic products however not canned ones plunged in syrup

• Grains like entire grains and refined grains. For instance, quinoa, oats, earthy colored rice, grain, and buckwheat

- Protein like lean hamburger and pork, chicken, fish, beans, peas, and vegetables
- Dairy items, for example, low-fat milk, yogurt, curds, and soy milk

A wide assortment for the determination of food decisions ought to be from every one of five nutrition classes in the particular sums suggested. These food sources from every nutrition type give a comparative measure of key miniature and full scale supplements to meet the body prerequisites.

A reasonable eating routine commonly contains 50 to 60 percent carbs, 12 to 20 percent protein, and 30 percent fat. Every one of the organs and tissues need legitimate sustenance to work actually by consuming the perfect proportion of supplements and calories to keep an optimal weight. The general wellbeing and prosperity of an individual are subject to great sustenance, actual activity, and sound body weight.

A legitimate feast design is a finished mix of food fixings, food things and amounts expected for breakfast, lunch, bite, and supper for every particular age bunch. All you want is

protein for your bulk and platelets which carries

oxygen and supplements to your muscles.

The body requires quality carbs, lean protein, fundamental fats and liquids joined by customary practice in keeping up with actual wellbeing and prosperity.

These are viable in forestalling abundance weight gain or in keeping up with weight reduction however better ways of life are likewise connected with further developed rest and temperament. Active work especially further develops cerebrum related capability and results.

Similarly as with active work, rolling out little improvements in your eating regimen can go quite far to achieve the ideal body weight. Consuming the right sort of starches is significant. Many individuals depend on the straightforward carbs tracked down in desserts and handled food varieties.

Products of the soil are rich wellsprings of normal fiber, nutrients, minerals, and different mixtures that your body needs to appropriately work. They're additionally low in calories and fat. Unsaturated fats might assist with diminishing aggravation and give calories.

The significance of a solid way of life

It's a reasonable eating routine that is enough as well

as sound acts of eating. Some of them which you can follow are:

• Eat-in more modest parts - You can do this by eating in little dishes to fool your mind into believing it to be bigger bits.

• Find opportunity to eat - Not surging your in the middle of between other work but rather carving out opportunity to support your dinners can convey messages to your cerebrum that you've had sufficient food vital for working.

• Eliminate snacks - Unfortunate tidbits are a severe no as they hamper your yearning. Changing to sound reduced down food can help.

• Check profound eating - Gorging can be very destructive. Utilizing it to ease yourself from stress, pity, or tension might influence your wellbeing. All things considered, you can

utilize better choices to beat
pessimistic feelings.

Chapter Three

Delicious Food You Should Avoid

Some foods are high in sugar, refined carbohydrates and fat, but low in essential nutrients such as protein and fiber. This can make it difficult to lose weight and have other negative health effects. Most people only focus on cutting calories to lose weight. However, it is also important to think about the foods you eat. Foods high in protein and fiber can keep you full longer, which can support weight loss

On the other hand, if you eat too many foods high in sugar, refined carbohydrates, or fat, you can add extra calories to your diet, making it harder to lose weight.

Here are 11 foods that can help you lose weight.

1. French fries and chips

French fries and potato chips are often very high in calories and fat. In observational studies, the consumption of

French fries and potato chips has been associated with weight gain and obesity. One 2011 study even found that potato chips can increase weight gain per serving more than any other food. In addition, baked, roasted or fried potatoes may contain substances called acrylamides, which have been linked to cancer. Therefore, it is best to enjoy these foods in moderation as part of a balanced diet.

2. Sugary drinks

Sugar-sweetened beverages, such as soda, are high in calories and high in sugar. They are strongly associated with weight gain and can have negative health effects if consumed in excess. Although sugary drinks are high in calories, the brain does not register them as solid food. Liquid sugar calories are not saturated, so you won't eat less food to compensate. Instead, you may need to increase those calories in addition to your normal intake. If you're serious about losing weight, consider cutting back on sugar-sweetened beverages in favor of beverages like flavored water, kombucha, tea, or coffee.

3. White bread

White bread is highly processed and often contains a lot of added sugar. It has a high glycemic index, which means it can cause a rapid rise in blood sugar. One 2014 study of 9,267 people found that eating two slices (120 grams) of bread a day was associated with a 40% greater risk of weight gain and obesity. Fortunately, there are many nutritious alternatives to conventional wheat bread, including Ezekiel bread, which is made from sprouted grains and legumes. But be aware that whole wheat bread contains gluten, which should be avoided by those with celiac disease or gluten sensitivity. Some other options for people on a gluten-free diet include opsi bread, corn bread, and almond flour bread.

4. Sweets

Confectioneries pack a large amount of added sugar, added oils and refined flour into a small package. Candy bars are also high in calories and low in nutrients. Many chocolate-covered candies contain about 200 to 300 calories, and extra-large bars can contain even more. For something sweet, consider a bite-sized candy bar or a few squares of dark chocolate and enjoy with other nutritious snacks like fresh fruit, nuts or a yogurt parfait.

5. Some fruit juices

Some fruit juices found in supermarkets have very little in common with whole fruit.

In fact, some types can contain just as much sugar and calories as soda, if not more. Also, fruit juice usually does not contain fiber and does not require chewing. This means that a glass of orange juice does not affect satiety in the same way as an orange, making it easier to consume large amounts in a short period of time. Opt for whole fruit instead or try to limit your fruit juice to about 118 milliliters at a time.

6. Pastries, cookies and cakes

Pastries, cookies and cakes are full of calories and added sugar. These foods are also not very satisfying, which means you can get hungry very quickly after eating these high calorie foods. If you are trying to lose weight, try to limit the portions of these foods and enjoy them occasionally as part of a varied diet. Foods like dark chocolate, fruit, trail mix or chia pudding can also help satisfy your sweet tooth.

7. Certain types of alcohol (especially beer)

Alcohol provides more calories than carbohydrates and proteins, about 7 calories per gram. However, the evidence for alcohol and weight gain is not clear

Moderate drinking looks good and is actually associated with less weight.

Heavy drinking, on the other hand, is associated with increased weight gain. The type of alcohol

is also important. Beer can cause weight gain, but drinking wine in moderation can actually be beneficial.

8. Ice cream

Besides being high in calories, most ice creams are also loaded with sugar. A small serving of ice cream is fine every now and then, but the problem is that it's very easy to consume large amounts in one sitting. Remember to serve yourself a small portion of ice cream instead of eating straight from the container so you don't eat too much. Alternatively, you can make frozen desserts using less sugar and nutritious ingredients like full-fat yogurt and fruit.

9. Pizza

Pizza is a very popular fast food. But commercially made pizzas are often high in calories and made with ingredients like highly processed flour and processed meats. If you want to enjoy a slice of pizza, try making it yourself at home using nutritious ingredients and toppings. If you're ordering from a restaurant, use low-calorie options like

roasted chicken, peppers, onions, spinach, mushrooms,

or garlic. You can also choose a thin-crust pizza to cut calories, or enjoy a slice or two of salad or steamed broccoli to round out your meal.

10. Calorie coffee drinks

Coffee contains several biologically active substances, including caffeine. These chemicals can boost your metabolism and increase fat burning, at least in the short term.

However, many coffee drinks contain too much cream and sugar, which can significantly increase the total calories in each serving. If you are trying to lose weight, it is best to limit your intake of these drinks or choose regular black coffee slightly sweetened.

11. Foods with a lot of added sugar

High consumption of added sugar is thought to contribute

to a number of chronic diseases, including heart disease, type 2 diabetes, obesity and liver disease. Foods high in sugar are usually high in calories, but lack other essential nutrients and are not very filling. Foods that may contain high amounts of added sugar include sugary breakfast cereals, granola bars, and low-fat flavored yogurt. You should be especially careful when choosing low-fat or fat-free foods, as manufacturers often add extra sugar to compensate for the flavor lost when the fat is removed.

CHAPTER FOUR

Nutritious Food You Should Eat More

Eating a wide variety of nutrient-dense foods, including fruits, vegetables, nuts, seeds, and lean proteins, can support your overall health. There are many healthy and delicious foods. Filling your plate with fruits, vegetables, high-quality protein sources, and other whole foods will give you a colorful, diverse, and healthy diet.

Here are 50 healthy and delicious recipes that you can incorporate into your diet.

1-6: Fruits and berries

Fruits and berries are

popular health foods. It's sweet, nutritious, and requires little to no preparation, making it easy to incorporate into your diet.

1. Apple

Apples contain fiber, vitamin C, and numerous antioxidants. It's very filling and perfect as a snack when you get hungry.

2. Avocado

Avocados, unlike most other fruits, are high in healthy

fats. Not only is it creamy and delicious, it's also rich in fiber, potassium, and vitamin C. Swap mayonnaise for avocado and use it as a salad dressing, or spread it on toast for breakfast.

3. Banana

Bananas are a good source of potassium. It is also rich in vitamin B6 and dietary fiber, making it practical and convenient to carry.

4. Blueberry

Blueberries are delicious and rich in antioxidants.

5. Orange

Oranges are known to contain a lot of vitamin C. Additionally; it is rich in dietary fiber and antioxidants.

6. Strawberry

Strawberries are highly nutritious and low in sugar and calories. It provides vitamin C, fiber and manganese and makes delicious desserts.

Other healthy fruits

Other healthy fruits and berries include cherries, grapes, grapefruit, kiwi, lemons, mangoes, melons, olives, peaches, pears, pineapples, plums, and raspberries.

7. Eggs

Eggs are very nutritious. Once demonized for their high cholesterol levels, experts now consider them to be a useful source of protein with a variety of benefits.

8-10: Meat

Lean, unprocessed meat can be incorporated into a healthy diet.

8. Lean beef

Lean beef is an excellent source of protein when consumed in moderation. It also provides highly bioavailable iron.

9. Chicken breast

Chicken breast is low in fat

and calories, but rich in protein. It is a great source of many nutrients.

10. Lamb and Mutton

Sheep are usually grass-fed and their meat tends to contain more omega-3 fatty acids than omega-6 fatty acids.

11-15: Nuts and seeds

Nuts and seeds are rich in unsaturated fats and calories, which can help reduce your risk of cardiovascular disease, cancer, and other health problems. A snack that is filling and helps with weight management. It also requires little preparation, making it easy to incorporate into your daily

routine. It can also add structure to salads and other dishes. However, it is not suitable for people with nut allergies.

11. Almond

Almonds are a popular nut containing vitamin E, antioxidants, magnesium and fiber. A 2021 study found that almonds can help with weight loss, support gut flora, improve thinking, regulate heart rate when under stress, and prevent skin aging. .

12. Chia seeds

Chia seeds are a nutritious addition to your diet. One ounce (28 grams) provides 11 grams of fiber and tons of magnesium, manganese, calcium, and a variety of other nutrients.

13. Coconut

Coconut provides fiber and fatty acids called medium chain triglycerides (MCTs).

14. Macadamia nuts

Macadamia nuts are delicious and contain more monounsaturated fat and less omega-6 fatty acids than most other nuts.

15. Walnut

Walnuts are highly nutritious and are rich in dietary fiber, various vitamins, and minerals. Combine with feta cheese and topping salads.

16. Brazil nuts

Brazil nuts are highly nutritious and have a smooth, buttery texture. The nutrients it contains support thyroid function and are an excellent source of the mineral selenium.

17-26: Vegetables

A calorie is a calorie, and vegetables contain the most concentrated nutrients. Including a variety of vegetables in your diet will provide you with a wide range of nutrients.

17. Asparagus

Asparagus is a popular vegetable that is low in carbohydrates and calories and rich in vitamin K.

18. Paprika

Bell peppers come in a variety of colors, including red, yellow, and green. Crunchy and sweet, they are a good source of antioxidants and vitamin C.

19. Broccoli

Broccoli is a cruciferous vegetable that is delicious both raw and cooked. It is a good source of dietary fiber, vitamins C and K, and contains a good amount of protein compared to other vegetables.

20. Carrot

Carrots are a popular root vegetable. It is sweet, chewy, and rich in nutrients such as dietary fiber and vitamin K. It is also rich in carotene antioxidants, which has many benefits. Include a few carrot sticks in your lunch box or use them to make guacamole or other dips.

21. Cauliflower

Cauliflower is a very

versatile cruciferous vegetable. It can be added to curries, roasted in olive oil, or used raw in salads and dips.

22. Cucumber

Cucumbers are a refreshing snack. It is low in carbohydrates and calories and consists mostly of water. It also contains small amounts of vitamin K and other nutrients.

23. Garlic

Garlic is a healthy and tasty addition to salads and cooked savory dishes. It contains allicin, which has antioxidant and antimicrobial effects. Its nutrients may also reduce the risk of cancer and cardiovascular disease.

24. Kale

Kale is rich in dietary fiber, vitamins C and K, and other nutrients. Adds rich flavor to salads and other dishes. You can also add it to fries or bake it in the oven to make crunchy kale chips.

25. Onions

Onions have a strong flavor and are included in many recipes. They contain many bioactive compounds that are believed to be beneficial to health.

26. Tomato

Tomatoes are technically a fruit, but they are usually classified as a vegetable. It's delicious and contains nutrients such as potassium and vitamin C. If you want to add a little fun and flavor, try growing tomatoes on your windowsill.

More healthy vegetables

Other vegetables worth mentioning include artichokes, Brussels sprouts, cabbage, celery, eggplant, green onions,

lettuce, mushrooms, radishes, pumpkin, chard, kale, beets, and zucchini.

27–32: Seafood

Fish and other seafood are healthy and nutritious. Rich in omega-3 fatty acids and iodine. Research shows that eating fatty fish improves heart and brain health.

27. Salmon

Salmon is a fatty fish that is delicious and rich in nutrients such as protein and omega-3 fatty acids. It also contains vitamin D.

28. Sardines

Sardines are small, oily, and highly nutritious fish. It contains many nutrients such as calcium and vitamin D.

29. Shellfish

Shellfish are highly nutritious and make for a light and delicious meal. Edible shellfish include mussels, mollusks,

and oysters. Be sure to get it from a trusted source to ensure it's fresh and toxin-free.

30. Shrimp

Shrimp is a type of crustacean similar to crabs and lobsters. They are usually low in fat and calories, but high in protein. It also provides selenium and vitamin B12.

31. Trout

Trout is also a delicious freshwater fish similar to salmon.

32. Tuna

Tuna is typically low in fat and calories and high in protein. Perfect for people who want to add more protein to their diet but need to keep calories low. Be sure to purchase low mercury varieties from responsible sources.

33-35: Grain

Whole grains play an important role in your diet because they are healthy carbohydrates and provide your body with a variety of micronutrients, fiber, and energy. It also helps with weight management.

33. Brown rice

Rice is a staple food for much of the world's population. Brown rice is more nutritious than white rice and is rich in dietary fiber, vitamin B1, and magnesium.

34. Oats

Oats provide a nutrient called beta-glucan and a

powerful source of fiber. Glucan has many benefits, including lowering cholesterol and nourishing the beneficial bacteria in your gut.

35. Quinoa

Quinoa is a delicious grain rich in nutrients such as dietary fiber and magnesium. It is also a good source of plant protein.

36–37: Bread

Whole grain bread is rich in

fiber and other nutrients and is a better choice than heavily processed white bread. When shopping for bread, compare product labels and look for products with the most dietary fiber and the least added sugar. When you bake your own bread, you know exactly what's inside. If you're not confident in making bread, a bread maker can help.

36. Ezekiel's Bread

Ezekiel's Bread is made from sprouted organic whole grains and legumes.

37. Homemade low-carb and gluten-free breads

If you're looking for low-carb or gluten-free breads, you might want to consider making your own. Here's a list of 15 recipes for gluten-free, low carb breads.

38–41: Legumes

Legumes are a great plant-based source of protein, iron,

and fiber. Legumes can sometimes interfere with digestion

and nutrient absorption, but soaking and properly preparing them can reduce this risk.

38. Green beans

French beans, also known as kidney beans, are an immature variety of the common kidney bean. Use as a side dish or chill and add to salads.

39. Kidney beans

Kidney beans contain dietary fiber and various vitamins and minerals. Cook properly as it is poisonous when raw.

40. Lens

Lentils are also a popular legume. It is rich in dietary fiber and is an excellent source of vegetable protein.

41. Peanuts

Peanuts are actually legumes,

not real nuts. They are tasty and high in nutrients and antioxidants. One study has concluded that peanuts can aid in weight loss and may help manage blood pressure. However, if you're monitoring

your calorie intake, you may want to be mindful of your consumption of peanut butter, which is very high in calories and easy to eat in large amounts.

42–44: Dairy

For those who can tolerate them, dairy products are a healthy source of various important nutrients.

42. Cheese

One slice of cheese contains about the same amount of nutrients as 1 cup (240 ml) of milk. It also makes a delicious addition to many dishes and replaces meat as a protein-rich food. However, it may contain a lot of fat. There are many types of cheese with different flavors and textures. Reduce the amount of processed cheese.

43. Milk

Milk contains vitamins, minerals, protein and calcium. A 2022 study concluded that people who consume dairy products are less likely to die from cardiovascular disease

than those who do not.

However, full-fat dairy products may increase your risk of cardiovascular disease and some cancers.

44. Yogurt

Yogurt is made by adding live bacteria to milk and fermenting it. Although it has many of the same health benefits as milk, yogurt with live cultures also has the added benefit of containing healthy probiotic bacteria.

45–46: Oils and fats

A diet containing unsaturated fats and oils is considered very healthy.

45. Extra virgin olive oil

Extra virgin olive oil is one of the healthiest vegetable oils. It contains heart-healthy monounsaturated fats and is rich in antioxidants with powerful health benefits.

46. Coconut oil

Although coconut oil is a saturated fat, it contains MCTs and may have similar health benefits as olive oil. However, coconut oil has been shown to raise LDL (bad) cholesterol levels more than other plant-based liquid oils. Therefore, it is best to use it in moderation.

47-48: Tuber

Tubers are storage organs in some plants. As a food, they are called root vegetables.

47. Potato

Potatoes provide potassium and contain almost all

necessary nutrients, including vitamin C. Potato skins are also an excellent source of fiber. Potatoes have higher water content and lower energy density than pasta or rice, making you feels full so you don't need to eat more. As a result, they may help with weight loss.

48. Sweet potatoes

Sweet potatoes are rich in antioxidants, beta carotene, vitamin A, and other essential nutrients. Eat them baked, mashed, or added to other dishes.

49. Apple cider vinegar

When taken with meals, apple cider vinegar helps regulate blood sugar levels after meals. However, more evidence is needed to prove its effectiveness. Ideal for dressing salads and seasoning dishes.

50. Dark chocolate

Dark chocolate contains

antioxidants called flavonoids, which may help control cholesterol levels and reduce your risk of heart disease. However, the amount of chocolate that is usually healthy is not enough to have any significant effect.

CHAPTER FIVE

Your Weight Loss Nutritious Plan

Dieting isn't just about losing weight. Changing your diet is one of the best ways to lose weight, but it can also be a gateway to improving your habits, taking care of your health, and living a more active lifestyle. However, with the vast number of diet plans available, it can be difficult to get started. Different diets are more appropriate, sustainable, and effective for different people. Some diets aim to suppress appetite and reduce food intake, while others recommend limiting calories and carbohydrate or fat intake. Some people focus on specific dietary or lifestyle changes rather than restricting certain foods. Additionally, many offer health benefits beyond weight loss.

Here are the 9 best diet plans to help improve your health

1. Mediterranean diet

The Mediterranean diet has

long been considered the gold standard for nutrition, disease prevention, health, and longevity. This is based on nutritional benefits and sustainability.

How to use

The Mediterranean diet is based on foods traditionally eaten by people in countries such as Italy and Greece. It is rich in the following:

- Vegetables
- Fruits

- Full grain

- Fish

- Nuts

- Lens

- Olive oil

Foods such as poultry, eggs, and dairy products should be consumed in moderation, and red meat is limited. Additionally, the Mediterranean diet has the following limitations:

Refined grains

Tran's fatty acids

Processed meat

Added sugar

Other highly processed foods

Health benefits

This diet, which emphasizes minimally processed foods and plants, is associated with lower risk of several chronic diseases and longer life expectancy. Research has also shown that the Mediterranean diet has protective effects against certain types of cancer (1).

Although this diet is designed to reduce the risk of heart disease, many studies suggest that a plant-based diet high in unsaturated fats may also help with weight loss (2). A systematic review that analyzed five different studies found that a Mediterranean diet led to greater weight loss after one year compared to a low-fat diet. Similar weight loss results were obtained when compared to low-carbohydrate diets (3). A 12-month study of more than 500 adults found that higher adherence to a Mediterranean diet was twice as likely to maintain weight loss.

Additionally, the Mediterranean diet encourages the intake of numerous antioxidant-rich foods that help fight inflammation and oxidative stress by neutralizing free radicals

Other benefits

Recent studies have also found that the Mediterranean diet is associated with a lower risk of mental health disorders such as cognitive impairment and depression.

Reducing meat intake also leads to a more sustainable diet for the planet. Cons

The Mediterranean diet places less emphasis on dairy products, so it's important to make sure you're getting enough calcium and vitamin D in your diet.

2. Dash diet

Dietary Approaches to Stop Hypertension (DASH) is a nutritional plan aimed at treating or preventing high blood pressure, clinically known as hypertension. The emphasis is on eating lots of fruits, vegetables, whole grains, and lean meats. It is low in salt and has added red meat, sugar, and fat.

Although the DASH diet is not a weight loss diet, many people report losing weight using it.

How to use

The DASH diet recommends specific portions of different food groups. The number of servings you are encouraged to eat depends on your daily calorie intake. For example, each day an average person on the DASH diet would eat about:

- Five servings of vegetables

- Five servings of fruit

- Seven servings of healthy carbs like whole grains

- Two servings of low fat dairy products

- Two servings or fewer of lean meats

In addition, it's recommended to consume nuts and seeds two to three times per week

Health benefits

The DASH diet has been

shown to reduce blood pressure levels and several heart disease risk factors. Also, it may help lower your risk of breast and colorectal cancers

Studies show that the DASH diet can also help you lose weight. For example, an analysis of 13 studies found that people on the DASH diet lost more weight over 8–24 weeks than people on a control diet

Another study in adults with obesity over 12 weeks found that the DASH diet helped decrease total body weight, body fat percentage, and absolute fat mass in study participants while preserving muscle strength

Other benefits

In addition to weight loss, the DASH diet may help combat depression symptoms

A comparative study over 8

years found that even moderate adherence to the DASH diet was related to lower depression risk

Downsides

While the DASH diet may aid with weight loss and lower blood pressure in individuals with hypertension, there is mixed evidence on salt intake and blood pressure. Eating too little salt has been linked to increased insulin resistance, and a low sodium diet isn't the right choice for everyone. Low-sodium diets like the DASH diet are suitable for people who have high blood pressure or other health

problems who would benefit from or require sodium restriction.

Further research is needed in this area to understand how a low-sodium diet affects insulin resistance in people without hypertension.

3. Plant-based and Flexitarian diets

Vegetarianism and veganism are the most popular variants of plant-based diets, which are limited to animal products for health, ethical, and environmental reasons. However, there are also plant-based diets that are more flexible, such as the flexitarian diet. This is a plant-based diet with a moderate intake of animal products.

How to use

A typical vegetarian diet restricts all types of meat, but allows dairy products. A typical vegan diet limits all animal products, including by-products such as dairy products, butter, and sometimes honey. Flexible meal plans don't include clear rules or recommendations regarding calories

and macronutrients, so

they're considered more of a lifestyle than a diet. Its principles include:

Get your protein from plants instead of animals

Eat mostly fruits, vegetables, legumes, and whole grains

 Eat foods that are minimally processed and in their most natural form limit sugar and sweets

It also provides the flexibility to consume meat and animal products at any time.

Health benefits

Numerous studies have shown that plant-based diets can reduce the risk of developing chronic diseases, including improving metabolic health markers, lowering blood pressure, and lowering the risk of type 2 diabetes. It also helps you lose weight

Additionally, a flexible diet has been shown to reduce the risk of type 2 diabetes and improve metabolic health and blood pressure.

Different advantages

For the people who are hoping to lead a practical way of life, diminishing your meat utilization can likewise lessen ozone depleting substance outflows, deforestation, and soil debasement

Drawbacks

Plant-based eating designs like vegetarianism and

veganism can in some cases be challenging to keep up with and may feel confining, particularly in the event that you're changing from a more meat-based eating style.

And keeping in mind that the adaptability of the flexitarian diet makes it simple to follow, being too adaptable with it might check its advantages.

4. The Brain diet

The Mediterranean-Run

Mediation for Neurodegenerative Deferral (Psyche) diet joins parts of the Mediterranean and

Run diets to make an eating design that spotlights on cerebrum wellbeing.

How it functions

Like the flexitarian diet, the Psyche diet doesn't have a severe feast plan, however rather energizes eating 10 explicit food varieties with mind medical advantages.

Each week, Psyche incorporates eating:

At least six servings of green, verdant vegetables

One serving of non-boring vegetables

At least five servings of nuts

Different food varieties it empowers on numerous occasions seven days include:

Berries

Beans

Olive oil

Entire grains

Fish

Poultry

Medical advantages

Research shows that the Psyche diet might decrease an individual's gamble of fostering Alzheimer's sickness, and studies show that the Brain diet is better than other plant-rich eating regimens for further developing insight

Research additionally shows that the Psyche diet can assist with easing back mental deterioration and further develop strength in more established grown-ups

It might likewise assist with postponing the beginning of the development issue Parkinson's illness

There is little exploration concerning the Brain diet and weight reduction. However, since a blend of two eating regimens advance weight reduction, the Psyche diet may likewise assist you with getting in shape.

One way it can assist with advancing weight reduction is that it supports restricting your utilization of food sources like:

Margarine

Cheddar

Red meat

Broiled food

Desserts

Nonetheless, more exploration should be finished

concerning the Psyche diet and weight reduction.

Different advantages

By joining the best of two weight control plans, the Psyche diet brings a great deal to the table and offers some more adaptability than stricter eating regimens.

While you can eat more than the 10 nutrition types it suggests, the nearer you adhere to the eating routine, the better your outcomes might be.

5. WW (previously Weight Watchers)

WW, previously Weight Watchers, is one of the most

famous health improvement plans around the world.

While it limits no nutritional categories, individuals on a WW plan should eat inside their set number of everyday focuses to assist them with arriving at their optimal weight

How it functions

WW is a focuses based framework that relegates various food varieties and refreshments a worth, contingent upon their calorie, fat, and fiber contents.

As you work to arrive at your ideal weight, you should remain inside your everyday point recompense.

Medical advantages

Many examinations show that the WW program can assist you with getting thinner

For instance, a survey of 45 examinations found that individuals who followed a

WW diet lost 2.6% more weight than individuals who got standard directing

Additionally, individuals who follow WW programs have been demonstrated to find success at keeping up with weight reduction following quite a long while, contrasted and the people who follow different eating regimens

Different advantages

WW permits adaptability, which makes it simple to

follow. This empowers individuals with dietary limitations, like those with food sensitivities, to stick to the arrangement.

Drawbacks

While it considers adaptability, WW can be expensive relying upon the membership plan and the time span you mean to follow it.

Concentrates on show that it might require as long as 52

weeks to deliver huge weight reduction and clinical advantages

Moreover, its adaptability can be a ruin in the event that calorie counters pick undesirable food varieties.

6. Discontinuous fasting

Discontinuous fasting is a dietary technique that cycle between times of fasting and eating.

Different structures exist, including the 16/8 strategy, which includes restricting your calorie admission to 8 hours out of each day. There's likewise the 5:2 strategy, which

limits your everyday calorie admission to 500-600 calories two times seven days.

While it's principally known

as an eating regimen for weight reduction, irregular fasting might have strong advantages for both your body and cerebrum.

How it functions

Irregular fasting confines the time you're permitted to eat, which is a basic method for decreasing your calorie consumption. This can prompt weight reduction — except if you remunerate by eating an excessive amount of food during permitted eating periods.

Medical advantages

Irregular fasting has been connected to hostile to maturing impacts, expanded insulin responsiveness, further developed cerebrum wellbeing, decreased irritation, and numerous different advantages

Both creature and human investigations show that discontinuous fasting may likewise increment heart wellbeing and broaden life expectancy,

It can likewise assist you with shedding pounds.

In a survey of studies, irregular fasting was displayed to cause 0.8-13% weight reduction over a time of 2 weeks to 1 year. This is a fundamentally more noteworthy rate than numerous different strategies

Different examinations found

that irregular fasting can increment fat consuming while at the same time saving bulk, which can further develop digestion

Different advantages

While specific weight control plans can have a great deal of rules, require continuous outings to the supermarket, and can be hard to follow, discontinuous fasting is known as an easier to-follow eating plan.

Because of the idea of the eating routine, there are fewer dinners that you want to plan, cook, and tidy up later.

Drawbacks

As a rule, irregular fasting is ok for most solid grown-ups.

All things considered, those delicate to drops in their glucose levels ought to converse with a wellbeing proficient prior to beginning discontinuous fasting. These gatherings incorporate individuals:

Who have diabetes?

Who have low weight?

Who have a dietary issue?

Who are pregnant?

Who are breastfeeding or chest feeding?

7. The Volumetric diet

The Volumetric diet was made by Penn State College sustenance teacher Barbara Rolls and is intended to be a drawn out way of life change instead of a severe eating regimen.

How it functions

The eating plan is intended to advance weight reduction by having you top off on supplement thick food sources that are low in calories and high in water.

In the interim, it limits calorie-thick food varieties like treats, confections, nuts, seeds, and oils.

The Volumetric diet separates food into four classes in light of food's calorie thickness, which can be determined with a recipe made by Rolls. These classes are:

Classification one: incorporates food sources of exceptionally low calorie thickness, as non-dull products of the soil, nonfat milk, and stock based soup

Classification two: incorporates low calorie-thick food varieties, as bland products of the soil, grains, breakfast oat, low fat meat, vegetables, and low fat blended dishes like bean stew

Classification three: incorporates medium calorie-thick food varieties, similar to meat, cheddar, pizza, bread, and frozen yogurt

Classification four: incorporates fatty thick food

varieties, similar to wafers, chips, chocolate confections, nuts, margarine, and oil

Feasts on the Volumetric eating regimen comprise generally of food sources from classifications one and two, with restricted measures of food from classes three and four.

No food varieties are totally untouchable on the volumetric diet, and exercise is energized for no less than

30-an hour every day.

Medical advantages

The Volumetric diet supports nutritious food varieties that are low in calories yet high in fiber, nutrients, and minerals, which might assist with expanding your admission of key supplements and safeguard against nourishing lacks

Research likewise interfaces eats less with a low calorie thickness to further developed diet quality

Also, it restricts how much handled food sources you'll eat, which can diminish your gamble of fostering specific tumors and coronary illness

The Volumetric diet may likewise assist you with shedding pounds.

A survey of 13 examinations in excess of 3,000 individuals found that eats less wealthy in low calorie thickness food sources prompted expanded weight reduction. Additionally, a 8-year concentrate on in excess of 50,000 ladies found that unhealthy thick food varieties prompted expanded weight gain

Drawbacks

While the Volumetric eating routine might be viable for medical advantages and weight reduction, it requires a decent comprehension of volumetric, which includes finding out about the calorie levels of food sources comparable to parcel sizes and supplement levels.

This might be simpler for some contrasted with others.

8. The Mayo Facility Diet

The Mayo Facility Diet was made by the trustworthy clinical association of a similar name.

How it functions

Intended to be a way of life

change over a handy solution, the Mayo Center Eating routine spotlights on supplanting less solid ways of behaving with ones that are bound to help life span and weight reduction.

Instead of forbidding specific food varieties, the Mayo Facility Diet utilizes a pyramid to support practice and represent amounts of food varieties you ought to devour.

Organic products, vegetables, and active work make up the foundation of the pyramid, trailed via carbs in the following layer, then protein and dairy, fats, lastly, desserts.

The eating regimen comprises of two stages. An underlying, 2-week stage intended to launch your weight reduction by presenting 5 better propensities and empowering you to bring an end to 5 normal less sound propensities.

The subsequent stage is to a greater degree a way of life change intended to be followed long haul, empowering training about nutritious food decisions and part measures as well as being truly dynamic.

Medical advantages

Little exploration is accessible about the medical advantages of the Mayo

Facility Diet.

In any case, the Mayo Facility advises clients to anticipate around 10 pounds of weight reduction during the initial fourteen days, and as much as 2 pounds during the subsequent stage.

Since consumes less calories wealthy in fiber can increment satiety by causing you to feel all the more full, the Mayo

Center Eating routine might

add to weight reduction. It might likewise diminish your gamble of creating type 2 diabetes

Furthermore, concentrates on show that practicing while on a lower-calorie diet is more powerful at advancing weight reduction than eating fewer carbs alone

Be that as it may, more examination is expected to decide the viability of the Mayo Facility Diet for weight reduction.

9. Low Carb Diets

Low carb eats less carbs are among the most famous weight control plans for weight reduction. Models incorporate the Atkins diet, ketogenic (keto) diet, and low carb, high fat (LCHF) diet.

A few assortments lessen carbs more definitely than others. For example, exceptionally low carb eats less carbs like the keto diet limit this macronutrient to under 10% of complete calories, contrasted and 30% or less for different sorts

How it functions

Low carb eats less carbs confine your carb admission for protein and fat.

They're commonly higher in protein than low fat weight control plans, which is significant, as protein can assist with checking your craving, raise your digestion, and preserves bulk

In exceptionally low carb slims down like keto, your body starts utilizing unsaturated fats as opposed to carbs for energy by changing over them into ketones. This interaction is called ketosis.

Medical advantages

Research proposes that low carb diets might diminish risk factors for coronary illness, including elevated cholesterol and pulse levels. They may likewise further develop glucose and insulin levels in individuals with type 2 diabetes

Many investigations show that low carb diets can help weight reduction and might be more successful than regular low fat eating regimens

For instance, a survey of 53 examinations comprised of 68,128 members found that low carb slims down brought about fundamentally more weight reduction than low fat eating regimens.

Also, low carb consumes less calories seem, by all accounts, to be very successful at consuming destructive tummy fat

Drawbacks

At times, a low carb diet might raise LDL (terrible) cholesterol levels. Exceptionally low carb diets can likewise be hard to follow and cause stomach related upset in certain individuals

In exceptionally uncommon circumstances, following an extremely low carb diet might cause a condition known as

ketoacidosis, a perilous metabolic condition that can be deadly whenever left untreated

CHAPTER SIX

Do Supplements Works

What Do Enhancement Do?

Whether they're pouring out of your medication cupboard or filling your washroom ledge, you're in good company on the off chance that you're one of the large numbers of Americans who take a nutrient or supplement every day.

You might be attempting to battle a lack of nutrient or lower your gamble of specific illnesses — - or you may simply have a proactive outlook on your wellbeing in the wake of popping an enhancement that vows to work on your wellbeing.

From vitamin A to zinc, Americans have been taking

dietary enhancements for quite a long time. At the point

when supplements previously opened up during the 1940s, individuals ran to neighborhood pharmacies to load up on these apparently otherworldly pills to work on their general wellbeing and prosperity — and they won't ever stop.

A Gander at Dietary Enhancement Utilization

Measurements

- More than 33% of Americans take supplements.

- Multivitamin or mineral enhancements make up 40% of all nutrient deals.

- The most widely recognized supplement contains fish oil, omega 3, DHA, or EPA unsaturated fats.

- Around 30% of grown-ups age 65 and more established takes at least 4 enhancements of any sort.

Dietary enhancement proposals can be found all over the place — on plugs, through web-based entertainment forces to be reckoned with, and from your neighbors, companions, and family. In the midst of the clamor, it very well may be difficult to tell which supplement — if any — is ideal for you.

However many enhancements are surely advantageous to your wellbeing, proof changes broadly, and it's essential to realize which can help your wellbeing and which might be hurtful.

5 Things you really want to be aware of Dietary Enhancements

1. Supplements come in

many structures.

"Whether in pill, powder or fluid structure, the objective of dietary enhancements is in many cases something very similar: to enhance your eating routine to get an adequate number of supplements and improve wellbeing," makes sense of Jeffrey Millstein,

MD, doctor at Penn

Interior   Medication
Woodbury Levels.

They contain no less than one dietary fixing, like nutrients, minerals, spices, botanicals, amino acids or proteins. Probably the most famous enhancements arrive in a multivitamin (which can assist you with trying not to take twelve pills every day), except they can likewise be bought as an independent enhancement.

The most straightforward shared factor? They're named as dietary enhancements. A few normal dietary enhancements include:

- Calcium

- Fish oil

- Echinacea

- Ginseng

- Garlic

- Vitamin D

- St. John's wort

- Green tea

2. Are supplements worth taking?

There's an explanation supplements are so well known: at times, they work.

"Notwithstanding a sound eating regimen, there is proof that a few enhancements can help your general prosperity with practically zero gamble," says Dr. Millstein.

Normal enhancements that might help your wellbeing

include:

• Vitamin B12, which can assist with keeping nerve and platelets solid, makes DNA and forestalls sickliness

• Folic corrosive, which can decrease birth absconds when taken by pregnant ladies

• Vitamin D, which can reinforce bones

• Calcium, which can advance bone wellbeing

- Nutrients C and E, which can forestall cell harm

- Fish oil, which can uphold heart wellbeing

- Vitamin A, which can dial back vision misfortune from age-related macular degeneration

- Zinc, which can advance skin wellbeing and dial back vision misfortune from age-related macular degeneration

- Melatonin, which can assist with neutralizing plane

slack

Nonetheless, regardless of how much examination that has been finished on supplements (starting around 1999, the Public Organizations of Wellbeing has spent more than $2.4 billion concentrating on nutrients and minerals), logical proof isn't totally clear. Remember: Most examinations recommend that multivitamins won't make you live longer, slow mental deterioration or lower your possibilities of infection, like coronary illness, malignant growth or diabetes.

"As a matter of fact, it's unlawful for organizations to make guarantees that enhancements will treat, analyze, forestall or fix illnesses," says Dr. Millstein.

Likewise, the items you purchase in stores or online might be not the same as those utilized in examinations, so studies might misdirect.

3. Supplements aren't protected all of the time.

Much of the time, multivitamins aren't probably going to represent any wellbeing gambles. All things considered, it's vital to be wary when you put anything in your body.

Dr. Millstein makes sense of, "Enhancements might collaborate with different meds you're taking or posture chances in the event that you have specific ailments, like liver sickness, or will have a medical procedure. A few enhancements likewise haven't been tried in pregnant ladies, nursing moms or kids, and you might have to play it safe."

Likewise, government guidelines for dietary enhancements are less severe than doctor prescribed drugs. A few enhancements might contain fixings not recorded on the mark, and these fixings can be dangerous. Certain items are advertised as dietary enhancements and really hold professionally prescribed drugs inside them — drugs that are not permitted in dietary enhancements.

A few enhancements that might present dangers include:

- Vitamin K, which can diminish the viability of

blood thinners

• Gingko, which can increment blood diminishing

• St. John's wort, which can make a few medications, for example, antidepressants and conception prevention, less compelling

• Natural enhancements comfrey and kava, which can harm your liver

• Beta-carotene and vitamin A, which can build the gamble of cellular breakdown in the lungs in smokers

4. Talk with your medical care supplier prior to taking any enhancements.

"The main thing to recall is to be savvy while picking an enhancement," says Dr. Millstein.

Your initial step ought to examine your choices with your medical care supplier, since an enhancement's viability and security might rely upon your singular circumstance and wellbeing.

What's more, remember these basic hints as you pick an enhancement:

• Accept supplements as coordinated by the name and your medical services supplier's directions.

• Peruse the name, including fixings, drug cooperation, and percent every day worth (% DV).

• Be careful about

outrageous cases, for example, "totally protected" or "works better than (embed doctor prescribed drug)."

• Recollect that the expression "normal" doesn't be guaranteed to approach "safe."

• Keep supplements put away appropriately and away from youngsters.

Find out about the expected risks of weight reduction supplements

5.   Nothing beats the supplement force of a sound eating routine.

Regardless of what your objective is while taking enhancements, one thing is sure: They aren't a trade for a supplement thick, sound eating regimen.

"Supplements are intended to be valuable — meaning they upgrade helps previously given by eating a balanced eating regimen," makes sense of Dr. Millstein.

Enhancements ought to never be utilized instead of genuine food. Try not to underrate how a supplement stuffed salad can help you contrasted with a pill made in a manufacturing plant.

Nutrients and minerals are fundamental for aiding your body creates and work as it ought to. All while a great many people get what's suggested by practicing good eating habits, others need some additional supplement help. That is where enhancements come in — giving you the help your body needs to remain solid.